Infertility Stinks!
By
Jacqueline Winslow

Infertility Stinks!

Table of Contents

Letter to the Reader

Day 1: It's Hopeless
Day 2: A Happy Mother of Children
Day 3: Praising God through the Storm
Day 4: Journaling
Day 5: Multiply Our Wombs
Day 6: Fear Not
Day 7: You Are Strong Enough
Day 8: Find Your Romance Mojo
Day 9: Dark, Dark Day
Day 10: Miracles and Angels
Day 11: God Loves You
Day 12: Ovulation Go-Getter
Day 13: Grace That Covers
Day 14: His Timing, Not Yours
Day 15: Do You Believe?
Day 16: True Surrender
Day 17: Fertility is My Portion
Day 18: Weary and Burdened
Day 19: Prayer
Day 20: Mind and Spirit Energizer
Day 21: True Love
Day 22: Jealousy
Day 23: Selfishness: Not Me???
Day 24: I am Hannah
Day 25: "I Can" Attitude

Day 26: Cramping Prayer
Day 27: Spread the Love
Day 28: "Life Messes"
Day 29: Dark Tunnel of Heartbreak
Day 30: Overcoming Miscarriage
Day 31: Infertility Prayer
Day 32: TTC Emotions

Scripture quotations are taken from New American Standard Bible (NASB) Copyright © 1960, 1962, 1963, 1968, 1971, 1972, 1973, 1975, 1977, 1995 by The Lockman Foundation

Letter to the Reader

In my journey of infertility, I came to a point in my life where I was overwhelmed, discouraged, and hopeless. To say I was fed up could have been the biggest understatement of the year. Life around me stood still, as if I were watching it pass me by.

Then, something unquestionably negative happened to me. I became ruthless, and I mean *ruthless*, in my TTC (Trying To Conceive) exploration. The incessant questions as to why I wasn't getting pregnant became a dark, hovering, tornado-like cloud that nearly consumed my life.

I knew I needed something to sustain me if I intended to continue our infertility journey. I began to soul search, and dug into my Scriptures. I finally managed to put my complete faith in Christ. I begin jotting down words of faith to help me through those many difficult moments. Pretty soon, my "infertility notes" became my own personal "infertility pocket devotional."

You see, the same thing happened every month: preparing for ovulation, ovulation, preparing for pregnancy, not being pregnant... etc... etc... etc... My life repeated itself like a broken record.

Ladies, infertility just stinks! It's emotional. It's heart-wrenching. It's financially draining. Did I mention it stinks? The pain, hurt, and frustration... the list could go on forever.

These emotions that are commonly felt throughout the month are real and we have to deal with them every single day.

For me, the infertility struggle happens minute by minute, hour by hour, day by day, and month by month. As I look back at my life, it becomes a blur of all the things we had to endure in our quest to get pregnant.

Does this sound familiar?

If so, you aren't alone. I feel it too.

Over the months and years, I came to the conclusion that infertility stinks! It just sort of happened. Infertility stinks! Well, actually, it came to me on one of those difficult days. Out of my mouth came the words that were the most fitting title for this devotional. I hope you can find little "faith nuggets" to help you through your own personal journey.

Our story may be different from yours, and our journey may be different too, but I am positive we share very similar emotions, thoughts, and hurts. These pages are what I go to when I need a smile, a renewed sense of hope, or a nugget of faith to continue the journey. There is hope!

You aren't alone.

With love and blessings,
Jacqueline Winslow
Our TTC (Trying To Conceive) Journey:
8 years,
100s of BFNs (Big Fat Negatives),
& 3 miscarriages

This devotional is dedicated to my true love.

Day 1: It's Hopeless

Then he said to me, "This is the word of the Lord to Zerubbabel saying, 'Not by might, nor by power, but my Spirit,' says the Lord of hosts.
Zachariah 4:6

The day is just beginning, and already I know it will be a tough one. Have you ever had that sense of foreboding of what is about to come? Maybe it's the Holy Spirit alerting us to pray. I hope so. Some days, we can feel the frustration, hurt, and disappointment before it ever comes. Somehow, we just know. It could be cramps, a false positive pregnancy test, or even signs of a miscarriage. On those days, it seems the hopeless emotions are trying to wage warfare with us.

It's not within our power. That should and can bring us relief. We don't have to walk this journey alone. Even more, we shouldn't because it can't happen through our power alone. How many infertility remedies have you tried that were unsuccessful? Or maybe you tried IVF, and still came up empty. Maybe you did everything you could find on the internet without a single pregnancy.

Be Fertile: It is good to know when nothing we do works, we can turn to our Savior. That hope reminds us we can overcome infertility. We can be fertile and have babies. Through Him, anything and everything is possible.

He makes all things new.

He makes the impossible, possible.

When your hope is gone, look up, and know that you can and will get through the day. Focus your eyes on God, not the situation. Pretty soon, the impossible starts to look actually possible. The truth is, we are looking at ourselves and our predicaments through God's eyes and not our earthly eyes. That simple, little nugget can help us through the darkest of days.

His strength will sustain us, and carry us.

God will give us hope and faith.

As we begin to lean on God for our hope and faith, we have to shut down the voices in our head. You know the ones. That little voice that often reminds you how many people have gotten pregnant. Or the one that repeats, *You aren't getting any younger*. And there's that other voice that just keeps screaming out, *Why God?*

I know! I have said those exact words about a hundred times a month. It's only natural when we see people all around us getting the one thing we long for – A Big, Fat, Positive Pregnancy Test! If you've ever wondered why you aren't getting pregnant, or why other women are getting pregnant, and not you, you can use those moments to say, *"It's not by my power and strength but by His spirit,"* says the Lord.

No matter how hard the day gets, you will make it through. It might seem difficult; His strength can and will get you through the darkest of days. On the day when you feel that cramp coming on, His strength will carry you through!

Don't be afraid; tell yourself, "I can make it. I will make it!" The dark day has to eventually end and morning always comes with a fresh ray of sunshine.

Let Him be your strength.

The truth is, life is never hopeless. It may seem like it, but it is never *hopeless*. THERE IS HOPE ETERNALLY. Despite how scared, frustrated, annoyed, angry, and every other emotion you can imagine, when we lift our eyes up toward the hill, where true help comes from, He will be there to give us the strength required to get us through whatever situation we face. We can put our hope in Jesus, and know He cares about our infertility.

Reflections

What situations can you release to God today?

What things do you need hope for?

Prayer: *Thank you, Lord, that it's through You. In this place, in this day, I choose to lift my eyes up to You, knowing you have my life in your control. Do big things in me today. Walk with me through this day. My hope is in You. My trust is in You. Be my strength. Be my hope. Be my faith. Do big things today in me, God. Amen.*

Notes:

_____

_____

_____

_____

_____

_____

Day 2: A Happy Mother of Children

He makes the barren woman abide in the house as a joyful mother of children.
Praise the Lord!
Psalm 113:9

Have you ever prayed, *God, please just let us have a baby?* or *When, God?* I know I often cried out those words. One year, I went to five baby showers in three months, and served as a baby coach! That summer was the longest and toughest of my life. Through it, however, I discovered a nugget that truly changed my life. Maybe you've had experiences just like that and said to yourself, "Not another baby shower!"

A pastor at the church we attended gave a sermon on being barren. His purpose was to show us how we can be barren in *life*. As I sat and listened to him quote Psalm 113:9, I knew I just received a huge chunk of faith, which I digested into my spirit. God cares about women struggling with infertility. He cares about the journey my husband and I must travel. God is interested in our miscarriages, our financial struggles, our IUI, and our plethora of infertility home remedies gone wrong. He cares about it all.

He settles the childless woman in her home as a happy mother of children.

God must have the perfect prescription to make any barren woman fertile. I certainly want that prescription, don't you?

Scriptures offer Hope, Faith, and Peace

I love Psalm 113:9 because it talks specifically about barren women. He is talking to us. God knows we need faith to get through each part of our journey. He knows we need hope to get through each day. He most certainly knows we need peace during the agonizing minutes in the bathroom spent while waiting for the pregnancy test to show + or -.

That peace provides the contentment to help us through whatever we must endure. We can be at complete serenity, trusting in God's plan and knowing we will eventually become mothers of children.

Take Steps of Faith

When we step out into faith and believe, He can make us happy mothers. We can be a family. We can hold that newborn in our arms, knowing our dreams have come true.

It's all about faith. Faith in what we cannot see. Anything is possible when we hold onto our faith and invest our trust in Him. The sky is the limit with God because His works are miraculous. That is what we need to hold onto.

God, I trust that you will make me a happy mother of children.

We want to see those miraculous works, don't we? How can we make it happen? We are, after all, struggling to conceive. We have to hold onto the promises God has given us! Believe and trust in Him, where anything is possible.

He settles the childless woman in her home as a happy mother of children.

Repeat this Scripture and believe it. Put it on a wall. Put it in your purse. Remind yourself often. God wants each of us to know he is concerned with our infertility struggle. Miracles can happen because He loves us and the children that are waiting to be born to us.

Reflections

What parts of this Scripture moved you?

Do you have the hope, faith, and peace to believe God will make you a happy mother of children?

Prayer: *God, I am a childless woman. Make me a happy mother of children. Take this barren body and make it fertile. On the bad days, give me miracles to remind me You are here. On the good days, give me miracles to remind me You are here. Let my life be a testimony of Your goodness. Make me a happy mother. Make me a mother, God. Amen.*

Notes:

_____

_____

_____

_____

_____

_____

Day 3: Praising God through the Storm

No temptation has overtaken you but as is common to man; and God is faithful, who will not allow you to be tempted beyond what you are able, but with the temptation will provide the way of escape also, so that you will be able to endure it.
1 Corinthians 10:13

Today, I am realizing how difficult it is to praise God. Another month spent waiting and hoping, is wearing down my faith. How do I choose to praise God on the good and bad days? Lately, I've had more difficult infertility days than good ones.

Today, when I can't see any signs of pregnancy, I have to accept the promise that God will not let me know yet. I choose to stand on His promise.

I have to dig deep in my heart, soul, and mind.

If I dig deeper than I ever thought possible, could God meet me there? Yes, God has met me there every time. God is always faithful to me when I dig deeply. When I think I have nothing left, He shows me the cap I set for myself isn't His limit for me. I can endure much more than I think I can. I am stronger than I realize or give myself credit for.

Do your thoughts center on all the things you've done in your quest for pregnancy? What can I try next? What new ovulation test or pregnancy test can I buy? Maybe you feel burnt out. Your strength is gone. Your hope is shattered. Your faith has become just a mustard seed in the wind.

> *Even here, in this hard place, can you turn your eyes toward the Great Comforter?*

Heartache: Failures, miscarriages, and negative pregnancy tests can thrust us into a dark spiral that feels like a never-ending roller coaster. Those dark thoughts can pull us down. Don't let heartache be your life song. Choose peace. Choose hope. Ignore the heartache. We all know what it feels like.

> *Your life Song can be Hope, Faith, and Peace!*

Somehow, we have to banish the "I can't get pregnant" thoughts and focus on giving God praise through it all.

> *We are alive.*

> *We have a happy marriage.*

> *We are blessed beyond measure.*

Choose to give God your praise. Give God the glory and thank Him for all you have. We can find peace, hope, and comfort when we turn our eyes toward God.

He will get you through every difficult situation, every time, and in every way. Hope and help await you. You and I have to simply reach out and grab what we need. He won't forsake us. When you think you can't go on any longer, God will give you the strength to take another step.

There were so many times in my infertility saga when I found myself at this exact spot. You know what? Every time, God gave me the courage to continue. You too will have the strength to endure.

Infertility Tip: Get away from the world. Get your Bible out and read your favorite Scriptures. You will be strengthened and encouraged. Post these Scriptures and words of faith around your house. Get sticky notes and repeat the Scriptures that speak most to you. They will help you!

Reflections

What storms are you facing today in your life?

Can you turn your eyes off the situation and rest your mind in Him?

Can you dig deeply inside of yourself and stand firm?

Prayer: *God, in my storm, help me turn my eyes toward you. No matter what happens in this infertility journey, I will keep my eyes, heart, spirit, and mind focused on You, oh Lord. Never let me forget you are right beside me. You are the true healer. Heal me, Father God. Thank you for never letting me down. Amen.*

Notes:

_____

_____

_____

_____

_____

_____

Day 4: Journaling

Bless the Lord, O my soul, And all that is within me, bless His holy name.
Bless the Lord, O my soul, and forget none of His benefits.
Psalm 103:1-2

I will say to the LORD, "My refuge and my fortress, My God, in whom I trust."
Psalm 91:2

Today I had a little miracle. In my home we call such things "toilet miracles." Do you know the kind of miracles I'm talking about? Do you remember a time where you prayed for something, whether small or big, and then, right out of the blue, it happened? Those are the best kinds of miracles, and I call them *toilet miracles.*

These small and seemingly insignificant miracles are the catalysts that propel us to bigger miracles. Write them down. Journal the miracles you don't want to forget. On those days when you are struggling with faith, pull out your journal and remind yourself of all those little miracles God provided for you. They may be *toilet miracles*, but they are still miracles: big or small makes no difference.

Praise the Lord for He is good. Reminding ourselves of what He has done for us is a great way to focus on the good and positive in our lives. God has done good things for each of us.
Our stories may be different.

Our miracles may be different.

But we are equally blessed, since God can do big things in our lives.

Whether they are *toilet miracles* or epic miracles, the more we look for them, the more miracles we will see. God is always working in our lives. The more we start to write down what God provides, the more faith we will have on those dark, hopeless days.

Big Days need Big Miracles.

Perhaps on the days when we test for ovulation, we need an extra big surge of faith and hope. Or maybe on the big day to test for pregnancy, we need those little reminders that the Lord is our refuge. We need the reminder that God is doing big things in our life. Our miracle journal will come in very handy on those dark days. I can assure you. I am a living testament to the big and small miracles God has done in my husband's and my lives. The key is looking for and recognizing them.

Infertility Tip: I know I need the Lord to be my refuge on those really difficult days. I know the rough days will come, but I have a plan of action in place. I grab a hot cup of my favorite fertility tea. I find a quiet place and journal all the ways God is helping my life. I focus on the good in my life. Some are about work. Some are about family. No matter what they are, or how different they may be for each of us: *Create a Miracle Journal.*

If you've never written a journal, now is as good a time as any to begin a new tradition. All you have to do is pull out a pen and notebook, and start writing. Write about your struggles and your miracles. The more you focus on the good, the more you will see. It's like awakening our eyes to all the good things happening in our lives. Through our struggles come the biggest miracles. How can we feel broken and beaten up after we read all the gifts God has bestowed on our lives?

Reflections

Do you have a toilet miracle?

What things has God blessed your life with today, big or small?

Prayer: *God, do big things today. Show yourself as a strong influence. Be my refuge through this process of getting pregnant. I need your strength. I need you in every way. Guard and protect my fallopian tubes and ovaries. Make them work properly. Let no evil come near me, my thoughts, my body, or my family. Protect me in every part of my life. Give me big miracles so that I can journal and remember all you've done for me. Amen.*

Notes:

_____

_____

_____

_____

_____

Day 5: Multiply Our Wombs

God blessed them; and god said to them, "Be fruitful and multiply, and fill the earth, and subdue it; and rule over the fish of the sea and the birds of the sky and over every living thing that moves on the earth."
Genesis 1:28

How many kids do you want? Are you praying for a full household? It's amazing how someone who struggles to get pregnant never cares how many kids they could have. They just want a child.

Give me a baby already! Please, I'll take one; just give me a baby, God.

If you've felt this way, you aren't alone. You are also not alone or abnormal when you lift your eyes up to heaven while praying those infertility prayers we've all prayed.

Be fruitful and multiply.

Thankfully, we can read and reread the stories where He endows the barren women with fertility. *Fertility* ... what a grand word it is.

God's wish is for our children to fill this earth. Guess what? You *are* fertile. When the doctor keeps telling you IVF is your only option, perhaps thinking you are fertile isn't high on your priority list. I get it. I've been there. So have many other women. Remember, God's ways are not our ways. Just because our eyes and ears hear one thing, that doesn't mean God doesn't have an entirely different plan – a miraculous kind of plan. Probably a special, God-sent fertility prescription where He says it's so and then it is. God is faithful and doesn't forget about you and me. He will bless our wombs.

We are fertile!

If you haven't seen the results yet, or anything that resembles a miracle, don't give up. Not only will God make us fertile, he will and can multiply our wombs. This Scripture is transforming. I read it daily to fuel the fire that builds within me. What we see as impossible is possible.

I choose to believe God will make me fruitful and multiply.

I choose to believe all things are possible.

Anything is possible to God! He can make your body work properly. Not matter what your problem is: PCOS (Polycystic Ovary Syndrome), blocked fallopian tubes, multiple miscarriages, or even a cold uterus – you can fill in the blanks. God can fix it or provide you with another plan to make it happen. I am a full believer in doctors and holistic approaches. However and whatever plan He gives you will be the right one.

Get ready for the bing, bang, boom! that has shaken me to my core. Even when the pregnancy tests say I'm not pregnant, I can hold onto the truth that God makes us fertile, and my day will come.

Whatever you do, giving up isn't an option.

Little by little, as you choose hope and faith, your faith will start to grow. It will fuel a fire within you. Whether you'd like to have one, two, or three kids, your faith will be like a volcano ready to burst.

Reflections

Do you believe God can make you fertile and multiply your womb?

Do you have a mustard seed of faith – because that's all it takes – just hold onto that mustard seed and let God cultivate it.

Prayer: *Oh, God, make me fertile. Multiply my womb. Remember your promise. Bless my womb so I can multiply. Fill my house with children. Give me faith so I don't give up when life gets really hard. Enlarge my faith. Enlarge my home. Make my body healthy. Heal my ovaries. Give me a fertility plan of action. Make my husband's body healthy. Give us a mighty miracle. Amen.*

Notes:

_____

_____

_____

_____

Day 6: Fear Not

For God has not given us a spirit of timidity, but of power and love and discipline.
2 Timothy 1:7

Today is a difficult and different sort of day. One minute life is good, the next, I am at the mercy of a tidal wave of emotions. It seems as if the emotions can cripple us in a second, because life is never easy.

Have you ever felt like that?

Have the fears of infertility pulled you into the depths of despair?

I am going to be very honest. I have moments where I am afraid. I am afraid God has forgotten about me. Afraid the months are going to drag into more years of nothingness. And then – the second I think I might succumb to my quiet, dreadful, downer thought, I remember the Scripture about not being afraid.

For God gave us a spirit not of fear, but of power and love and self-control.

My spirit refuses to harbor fear. I mentally proclaim: God gave me power and self-control. I choose to not be afraid of my circumstances. I take control of my thoughts, my quiet, downer thoughts, and choose prosperity. I choose hope. I choose obedience. I choose to fear the Lord rather than fearing the issues of my life.

Power, love, and self- control direct us toward a Christ-centered life. As a result, the more we control our thoughts, the more power we have over the dreaded fears.

When we choose to allow fear to creep into our minds, we aren't fully walking in the path God intended for us. Our hidden and known fears can be the very obstacles that stop us from embracing God's promises. Here's just a small list of possible fears:
- Fear of failure
- Fear of the inability to conceive
- Fear of never holding your own baby
- Fear of being motherless
- Fear of miscarriage
- Fear of inadequacy
- Fear of man
- Fear of being alone

Those are just a few in a long line of fears than often try to grip us during our journey to conceive. I'm sure you could add your own fears to this list. Please do. Add whatever fears that immediately come to your mind. Those are the fears you want to manage and take control of.

Your fears can precede a spiral of emotions that often lead you into a dark hole. Basically, when we allow our fears to consume us, we shut God and the world out. His blessings are just a fingertip away, but our fears can be substantial stumbling blocks.

Fear does not come from God. God whispers life into each of us. If you feel fear coming on, focus on your faith rather than the fearful thoughts. The worry of being infertile can be all encompassing, not to mention, repeating a miscarriage, or whatever other fear exists. They are real. However, God's grace as we turn our eyes back to Him will ease our fears until they exist no more.

Reading Scriptures Can Turn Fear into Hope and Faith

Using self-control and the power to NOT indulge fear often makes us fall back on our knees as we cry out for God to hear us, see us, and move in us. The more we live a Christ-like life, the more we focus on what God can do, instead of what we consider lacking in our lives.

Our worst fears can become the catalysts for what makes us the most faithful. Instead of being afraid of failure, we can lift our chins and refuse to let those fears consume us. His love is sufficient for us. He gives us self-control and power. We *can* choose to not be afraid of the unknown. We *can* choose faith. Fear can't control us if we don't allow it.

Reflections

What are your fears?

Are you afraid of never getting pregnant?

Can you release that fear, and trust that God has you safely in the palms of His hands?

Prayer: *God, give me the strength to face each day free of all fear. Encourage me when I am at the lowest of lows. Bless me today and remind me that You only want good things for me. Bless us with children. Take my fears and turn them into faith, hope, and joy. When my fears feel like they are overtaking me, give me words of hope and faith. Remind me of Scriptures to get me through my day. Send me miracles to remind me You are here. Amen.*

Notes:

_____

_____

_____

_____

Day 7: You are Strong Enough

"Have I not commanded you? Be strong and courageous! Do not tremble or be dismayed, for the Lord your God is with you wherever you go."
Joshua 1:9

Have you ever had something happen and only after the situation was over, found it hard to believe you survived? You did it. You had the strength and fortitude, even when you thought you had nothing left! You made it through the worst situation; and you survived.

Infertility is easily one of the most difficult circumstances a couple can face. After months of IVF, artificial insemination, ovulation tests, pregnancy tests, and shots, life for women dealing with infertility can seem challenging, painful, and fearful.

Be strong and courageous.

How is it that no matter what we must endure, we somehow find the courage to make it through? Despite the most difficult obstacles, you and I manage to muster the courage to dig deeper and muddle through even the hardest of situations.

Right now, in this place, you must know this: you will make it through. Whatever your "life situation" is, you will make it to the other side. No matter how difficult it may seem, no matter how much pain you are going through, you are not alone.

God will be with you wherever you go.

When life gets tough and we're honest, really honest, with ourselves, that is when we need to remember:

God is with us, and we are strong enough.

Put one foot in front of the other foot and keep going. You can do it. You will make it through whatever ordeal you are currently going through. Don't be afraid. You aren't alone. God is always with you. If you have no strength left, if it all seems depleted, and you are exhausted, remember this passage:

Have I not commanded you? Be strong and courageous. Do not be afraid; do not be discouraged, for the LORD your God will be with you wherever you go.

You see, although infertility may be a whopper of a problem we must deal with, we all know life can throw us even larger lemons. The lemons can take many different forms.

TTC (Trying to Conceive) is just one overripe lemon we, as women, must deal with; although, I'm sure, you could list off a dozen or more. God knows we are strong enough. He knows we will find the necessary courage. Whatever your "lemon" is, you will overcome it.

We all know what to do when a large, sour lemon comes our way, don't we? Yes, we may want to vent, cry, scream, kick, and even throw a tantrum. I'll be honest with you, I've wanted to do each of the things listed more than once during my infertility journey. Anyone reading this who has struggled to get pregnant knows just how brutal life can be. Can I get an Amen here, ladies?

What happens after we've spent our last emotion?

We did deeper and know we can make it through whatever comes our way. He will never give us too much to handle. We can dig deeper – God will give us the strength and courage to face life's lemons with grace, courage, and integrity.

It might take a lot of prayers before we discover a part of us we didn't even know existed. Prayer works! You see, we are strong enough. The Bible reminds us over and over of this. We are brave enough. We do have enough faith. Remember the mustard seed? Dig deeper and hold onto that mustard seed of faith.

The key is to reach out, and grab hold of it. You can't see it, but you can feel it. Faith, hope, courage, strength - all of these attributes are attainable, and accessible, right when problems happen. In the second a problem arises, if we pray, and have patience, while holding onto our faith, we can watch and see what God will do. It's that easy.

Infertility Tip: Sometimes it requires us to lay down our burdens, stop thinking about them, and focus on Scriptures. Did I mention patience? Get ready, ladies, because you might just need more of it. Take those lemons and make some fresh, sweet lemonade!

Reflections

What areas of your life do you need to be courageous in?

Are you discouraged in your infertility journey?

If so, can you take the lemons and make sweet lemonade?

Prayer: *God, show me my courage. I can do this. Help me believe that I am strong enough. Through You, I am strong enough. No matter what comes my way, You will give me the strength and fortitude to deal with every lemon that comes my way. You are greater than my infertility and every other problem in my life. Through You, nothing will occur that I can't handle. I am strong through You, God. God, I need strength, I need hope to make it through this infertility process. The days are long and hard. Some days, I just don't think I can handle anymore. Help me be strong and courageous. Some days, I am afraid and discouraged. Help me on those days. I want to have faith and hope. Be with me God, I need You. Amen, Amen, and Amen.*

Notes:

_____

_____

_____

Day 8: Find your Romance Mojo

Hatred stirs up strife, but love covers all transgressions.
Proverbs 10:12

May he kiss me with the kisses of his mouth!
For your love is better than wine.
Song of Solomon 1:2

For me, my marriage is my happy place. I think of it as my zen retreat where I go when I need strength. In a happy world, it's all perfect. Sadly, that isn't the case as soon as infertility enters the picture. The stress of trying to conceive unsuccessfully can be taxing on you and your marriage. If there is any nugget I could impart to you, it is to find your romance mojo, and use it often. A happy marriage will sustain you through all the obstacles life happens to cast your way.

If you're wondering what romance mojo is, think of it as a secret spark between you and your spouse. It's a safe haven that only you two know about. It's that "thing" that makes you giggle like a school girl, and stokes the fire that ignites from a simple wink he gave you.

Romance is Sweeter than Candy

Romance is indeed sweeter than candy. Come on, girls, let's be deep. When you find that happy place with your true love, everything just feels better. Romance is like your favorite chocolate with whipped topping. Find the special mojo and it will keep your marriage happier than ever. You know what works for you and your true love. Find it and go there often.

It can happen no matter how many years you've been married. Remember the old saying, "It only takes two to tango?" It all begins with true love. From there, write a love story that belongs to you and your love alone. Create a timeless love story. It's a never-ending love story you get to create. From there, relive your love, rediscovering your romance, and enjoying why you fell in love.

Kiss me and kiss me again...

I think I need to pause here and go find my true love...

If I was you, I would do the same...

Emotional Exhaustion: The truth is, after months of trying to conceive, it can drain you. It's very exhausting. Who wants to think about romance after months of trying to conceive? It's fertile week once again; and it's going to be 1-2-3. You know what I mean. There's a cycle and this girl is going to follow it. Who has time to think about romance? All I can think about is: charting my cycle, ovulation sticks, cervical mucous and a hundred other issues. Um, if this is you, keep reading!

Infertility can exhaust you, your spouse, and your marriage.

Let's face the facts, girls, we can get OCD over fertility and getting pregnant. Life can become more about automated "love times," than spending time loving our husbands. Pretty soon, we are stressed, worn out, and fighting with our spouses. Does that sound familiar? If so, you need to do one important thing this month:

Forget about getting pregnant.

Say what? Yes, I did say *forget about getting pregnant.* The more we focus on getting pregnant, the more stressed out we can become. We can and should focus more on romance, communication, and the little things in life. Hey, I'm not saying to forget about your cycle and what days are the + days. I'm just saying to reestablish your romance and find the romance mojo. We need that safe place where we can run. For me, my safe haven is, always and forever, my husband.

Tips for Finding Romance Mojo:

Hold hands for no good reason.
Kiss in the middle of the store.
Hold hands while you lie in bed.
Write a love letter.
Be selfless.
Be encouraging.
Do something unexpected.
Go on a date.
Prepare a romantic dinner/movie.
Whisper sweet nothings to him.
Wink for no reason.

Whether you whisper sweet nothings in his ear, or giggle your way to the bedroom, the point is to rediscover love in every moment of your day. Be the first one to step up to the plate.

Small moments can turn into passionate romance novels.

It's possible, one little kiss at a time.

Reflections

How can you focus on romance today?

What little things can you do for your spouse to add unexpected romance to his and your day?

One little kiss, one big kiss, one little kiss, one big kiss – repeat and try again.

Prayer: *God, help us enhance our marriage. Don't let infertility and our attempts to get pregnant take away from what we already have. We want this baby more than life itself. Please turn our struggles into our greatest joys. Help us to rediscover romance in the middle of hardship. Bless my marriage. Bless my spouse. Enlarge our family. We need You in our life. Help us give of ourselves freely and selflessly. Give us passion. Redefine our marriage. Amen.*

Notes:

_____

_____

_____

Day 9: Dark, Dark Day

Then they cried to the Lord in their trouble.
And He brought them out of their distresses.
He caused the storm to be still,
So that the waves of the sea were hushed.
Then they were glad because they were quiet,
So He guided them to their desired haven.
Let them give thanks to the Lord for His lovingkindness,
And for His wonders to the sons of men!
Psalm 107: 28-31

Dark days may enter your life. Sadly, it's a part of the journey of life. On those days, trust that He will calm the storms that arise. When the storm blusters, immediately look up to Him. The Lord will bring you out of your distress, whatever that may be. When the darkness begins closing around you that is when you and I have to lift our eyes, our thoughts, and our emotions up to God. Cry out to the Lord. Tell him what you are feeling, needing, and wanting. Talk to God like He is standing right beside you.

Yes, push away any thought that doesn't come from Him. If you can push it all away, and give thanks to the Lord, He will calm the storms in your life.

Our Storms Can Turn into Miracles!

When we cry out to the Lord, our belief and faith open the door to so many good things – like miracles! Sometimes, there will be dark days only you and I can imagine when all we have the strength to do is:

Cry Out The Name of Jesus.

Perhaps your period has begun, and the cramping hit you like fireworks. Your emotions are on a roller coaster. Here, in that critical moment, is when you say:

I praise You, Jesus, through this storm. This may be a dark day right now, but I'm going to lift my eyes to You. I will rejoice no matter how bad I feel."

Walking in faith is all you need to do. We don't have to see it to believe it. Cry out to the Lord in your hour of trouble and despair. He, alone, can still our raging storms. Let our tears turn to praise for Him. When we cry out to God at times when we feel the worst, we can anticipate our excitement because we know God is about to move. He will move to bring us out of our distress.

*They were glad when it grew calm,
and he guided them to their desired haven.*

Reflections

In any storm you encounter, choose prayer first.

Whether short or long, prayers can become miracles in your life. The storms in life will come eventually, so be prepared. Prayer, faith, and praise can be life-changing.

Prayer: *God, help me lift my eyes, heart, emotions, and thoughts up to You in my dark days. When I have nothing left to give, help me turn to You so You can do miraculous things in my life. God, I need miracles. Still the storm in my life so that Your will can be fulfilled. Guide us to a haven where we can find comfort through our struggles. Amen.*

Notes:

_____

_____

_____

_____

_____

Day 10: Miracles and Angels

For it is written, "He will command His angels concerning You to guard you." Luke 4:10

And He said to them, "Because of the littleness of your faith; for truly I say to you, if you have faith the size of a mustard seed, you will say to this mountain, 'Move from here to there,' and it will move; and nothing will be impossible to you.
Matthew 17:20

Do you need a new supply of hope to keep going? Is there a mountain you need to have moved? Get ready; today's devotional is about the supernatural, miracles, and angels.

Nothing is impossible with God.

Imagine this: you're struggling with infertility. One morning you are praying, and God gives you a new plan of action. You follow this plan. Many months later, you become pregnant. That is the power of prayer. For many people in the Bible stories, that was exactly what happened. God gave them a plan of attack, which they followed, and the miracles ensued.

All we need is a mustard seed of faith.

The possibilities of what God can do in our lives are endless. He not only sends angels to guard and protect us, but he can also move any mountain blocking our path!

God's Angels: Did you know God has angels looking out for you as you prepare for pregnancy? For each step you take, God has guardian angels to watch over you. Just as you take prenatals, or do that daily fertility massage, drink your fertility tea, or do IVF – no matter what you have to do, you aren't alone. God's angels are singing over you.

Visualize this: the heavens rejoicing as the eggs and sperm travel down the fallopian tubes. Can you hear the sounds now? I can. They are rejoicing, praying, and urging the miracles to happen. Knowing that God has ordered his angels to protect and guard us should compel us to have more faith. God cares about protecting our wombs, our health, and fulfilling our lives… now, isn't that something to get excited about?

If we have angels looking out for us, there is more hope for my miracle, your miracle, and our miracles.

What Has God Done in Your life?

Take a moment to think about you, your life, and all God has done for you. Think about those times when something out of the ordinary happened. Like a time you were in need of something and it suddenly appeared. Did you pray? It might not have been an immediate miracle. I've seen prayers answered in days, weeks, months, and even years. What prayers have you had answered? Do you remember them detail for detail?

I choose to believe that God sends his angels to watch out for me. I choose to have faith to believe the mountains in my life will be moved.

Reflections

Do you have a mustard seed of faith? If so, that's more than enough!

Thank you, God, for the angels watching over my body.

Prayer: *God, I acknowledge every miracle You have done in my life. Thank You for showing me how much You love me, my life, and my fertility journey. I'm thankful for those angels that are watching out over me. When I'm weak, replant that mustard seed of faith to keep me going. Amen.*

Notes:

_____

_____

_____

_____

_____

_____

Day 11: God Loves You

For God so loved the world, that He gave His only begotten Son, that whoever believes in Him shall not perish but have eternal life.
John 3:16

    The day is over. My work is done; dinner is fixed; and I'm ready for bed. As I lean against my husband in utter exhaustion, I can't restrain my smile. I am putting myself through misery with the Clomid, but I cling to one thing - it will be worth it!

    Somehow in these moments, I feel God's love all around me. To think He sacrificed his only son for you and me, even now, still leaves me speechless. I'll be honest, through my Clomid months, I've had many moments spent in the depths of despair. Those moments, however, can't last long because faith quickly overtakes my thoughts. God is too immense and He loves us too much. If you struggle with infertility, you may have experienced some of those moments too. Today, find a place away from the rest of the world. Tell yourself out loud how much God loves you.

God cares about what happens to you.

    The knowledge that God loves us serves to remind us that we will get through whatever the day brings. There is hope for tomorrow. God's love will shine down like the sun. His love is like a beautiful rainbow after a terrible storm.

The storm may come, but never lasts. Just hold on. Hold onto the promises He's given you.

Infertility Tips: My favorite way to get through infertility struggles is what I call my "infertility playlist." When I feel worn out, I go straight to the Christian music that invariably lifts me back up. I find hope, faith, and peace every time.

Reflections

God loves you. You are precious in God's sight. Enough said.

Prayer: *God, thank You for your love. Thank You for loving me enough to sacrifice Your Son for my sins. Help me feel Your love on those days when I need it the most. Some days, I feel so defeated. On those days, give me flowers of hope. Lift my spirits when I need it most. Send me reminders that I need quiet time with You. Remind me You love me. Amen.*

Notes:

_____

_____

_____

_____

_____

_____

Day 12: Ovulation Go-Getter

For You formed my inward parts;
You wove me in my mother's womb.
Psalm 139:13

Then Jesus said to her, "O woman, your faith was great; it shall be done for you as you wish." And her daughter was healed at once.
Matthew 15:28

Before we begin today's devotion, let's take a few minutes to escape from all the challenges of the world. Whatever is going on in your life: work, your husband, getting pregnant, or finances, just relax, take a deep breath, and exhale out all your frustrations. Take another long breath, no matter how stupid it sounds. It does work; as you let out your breaths, let go of whatever is resting on your shoulders.

It is going to be okay, ladies.

You will make it to the other side of whatever obstacles are in front of you. The "whatever" might be different for each of us, but we know for certain that through Christ, we can make it through ANYTHING. Hold on.

Today it's all about pumping you up. This isn't a normal day. This is THE DAY you've been prepping for - ovulation.

Today is all about faith. It's the day you need faith the most. These are some of my favorite "Fertility Go-Getter Phrases," which I lean on when days get hard. Use them. Better yet, create your own Fertility Go-Getter Phrases. You can do this. You are more than a conqueror. Get your fight song on, and be ready to take leaps of faith.

- God, give me a Hannah moment.
- I am fertile.
- Infertility is just an opportunity for God to do a miracle in my life.
- I have a mustard seed of faith. God, move in me.
- Bless my womb, God.
- When I get discouraged, give me miracles to remember, God.
- Fertility is an opportunity for extra romance.
- Trying to conceive helps me put God first. I put You first in my life, God.
- There is power in prayer.
- I have angels looking out for my womb. I can be at peace.
- I choose to fear not. I will not fear the inability to get pregnant. I choose faith!
- Fertility is my potion.
- I will be a happy mother of children. I will not be childless for long. God will save the day.
- I will NOT give up. I won't let myself stop believing. I will believe. I will have hope. I choose faith.
- The Lord is my rock and my shield. I will trust in my Lord, my God.
- God is my rock and my fortress; whom shall I fear?
- Yes, Lord.

- I will trust in the Lord, my God.
- I will guard my words and thoughts. I will think before I speak.
- Infertility requires that we dig deep as the path can be long and hard.
- When I hear negativity, I will breathe deep and remember: unless they've been in my shoes they just can't understand. I will hold onto my dream.
- Giving up isn't an option.
- I can get back up and try again. There is success in trying.
- I am not a failure. Just because I haven't gotten pregnant yet, I can and will keep trying.
- There is power in having faith in my life, no matter what happens.
- How great is my Savior God! My God is all-powerful to hear every prayer I pray.
- I will dig deep when life throws those angry darts my way.
- I've got to be quiet and retreat to my prayer closet. Prayer moves mountains.
- God is in control over my life. He sees what I can't.
- Can't is not a word in my vocabulary.
- When I've had all I can handle, I need "Me and God time."
- A negative pregnancy test is just another reminder my miracle isn't here yet, but it *is* coming. I just have to hold on a little longer.
- Sometimes, prayer is the only thing that can help our emotional wounds. Prayer and waiting on the Lord. He will renew our strength.

- Remember, tomorrow is always fresh with no mistakes or failures in it. The dawn will come and bring new hope for a better day.
- As rain falls outside, let this be a reminder and prayer for God to pour blessings over me. Send blessings in my life body, and my heart. Let the rain remind me that God will pour out His blessing over me. Send the rain, God.

Reflections

I choose words of faith today. I believe I am more than a conqueror today.

I am fertile.

My ovaries are working properly. My fallopian tubes are healthy and clear.

I believe.

I will make it through this.

Prayer: *How great is our God! Give us a big miracle today. Do big things in us. I am looking for a big, fat, miracle, God. I am walking in faith, and standing strong. I am keeping my eyes lifted to heaven. I know You are a miraculous God. Be miraculous in my life. Whisper words of hope to me when I need them most. Help me keep my faith strong. I can do this, God, with Your help. I need You. Amen.*

Notes:

_____

_____

Day 13: Grace That Covers You

For of His fullness we have all received, and grace upon grace.
John 1:16

Grace and peace be multiplied to you in the knowledge of God and of Jesus our Lord.
2 Peter 1:2

I'll be honest. During my Clomid months, I fell into the depths of despair quite a few times. If you struggle with infertility, you must have had those moments too. And that deep longing that never sees the light of day. Grace, I need you, kinda moments. Sometimes they come by the hour, and sometimes by the minute.

Fertility drugs are brutal. Their side effects are vile. Especially if you are the type of woman who gets every side effect listed on the bottle. I am just that woman. It's in this place, when I need God's grace. And the moment I realized I was having a miscarriage, I needed God's grace. It is when I look into my husband's eyes and see how badly he yearns for a baby. I need God's grace.

Have you had those horrible days when all you can do is cling to that tiny shred of hope that it will be worth it one day? And all the effort you put in will pay off eventually? The good news for every woman struggling with infertility is – grace will comfort us when we need it most. Grace and peace are ours for the taking. No matter how bad your month gets, grace is right there to help us meander our way through life. His grace will comfort us no matter how desperate we might feel.

Grace is like a big cloud that follows you wherever you go. The rain falling down on you is like continual grace for all life's struggles. All we have to do to receive God's grace is ask for it. Grace flows over us because God loves us and knows our needs better than we do. He douses the right amount of grace on us.

God, give us grace today.

Sometimes, leaning into God's love and grace may be as simple as just shutting off your thoughts - getting quiet and asking Him for grace. I need lots of grace. Whether on the days I ovulate, or the days I expect my period. There is no point through the month that we can't appreciate an abundance of grace.

As soon as you ask for grace, it's there. My mom always used to tell my sisters and me to breathe deeply. Although we shrugged off her words with laughter as kids, the talent of breathing in and out is a good habit that each of us need to master. Breathe in, long and slow, and breathe out all your hurts, pains, and frustrations. Try this every day and you will be amazed how much it helps. Breathe and pray!

Reflections

In what areas do you need grace today? No matter what you need, God will be there.

Just ask. Don't be afraid to talk to God as your father.

He is always there, and listening to you.

Prayer: *I need Your grace to cover my life, my finances, my emotions, my marriage, and my womb. This journey is hard, God, and I need Your help. My tears fall freely as my emotions overtake me more than I want to admit. You know though, God. You know my thoughts, and my dreams of a baby. You know how I cry when I see other women holding their newborns. You know how I cry in the bathroom when I realize I'm not pregnant – again! You know God. Help me lay it all down. Help me manage my desires. I need You, God. Amen*

Notes:

_____

_____

_____

Day 14: His Timing, Not Ours

He has made everything appropriate in its time, He also set eternity in their heart, yet so that man will not find out the work which God has done from the beginning even to the end.
Ecclesiastes 3:11

It's His timing, not ours. What a nauseous thing to even say out loud. It's one of those times when I can't believe I'm actually saying it; but I know it's true. Our lives truly are in God's hands.

Do you get emotional talking about your infertility journey? I mean, really getting open about the subject? It could be how you feel when you are sitting on the toilet with a pregnancy test in your hand. Or maybe it's that moment when the cramps start; how do you feel in that very second?

You see, infertility is an emotional subject. I dread the moment when someone comes up to me and says, "It's all God's timing, honey."

We know it's all God's timing, don't we? We live it. Don't need to tell us about timing.

Can I get a witness, ladies?

How many of you, like me, have thought all too clearly what we would have liked to say back to that person? As if we didn't think already, long and hard, about why God was taking His sweet time – of course, we know we have to wait on God. That's a no-brainer.

Just because we know it doesn't mean it's easy to digest.

God never said our Christian walk would be easy.

Life isn't easy.

That much we all know to be true. The uneasy parts of our lives are the times when we really have to let loose, and say, "God, you have control of my life." That means, our desires are governed by His timing. We want His timing. No matter how long we've waited, God always knows best.

He's never failed us yet. He won't fail us as we combat infertility. If we can hold onto the little *toilet miracles* during these times, how much greater will the bigger miracles seem when they happen?

God, You have full control of my life.

Say it often, and repeat it to yourself. On those days when nothing is going right, repeat it. God does have control. He will take care of you. He does know what he is doing – even when your wait seems like a long time. We might not get pregnant when *we* want to, but that doesn't mean God doesn't have a plan for us. He does! He has a perfect plan for us and we just have to walk in faith. We can do it.

Remember, faith is not seeing, but believing. Believe with your heart that God can make you a happy mother of children. Belief begins with a mustard seed. Grab hold of that mustard seed and believe in the God of miracles. He can create any miracle for us.

God's Timing is Always Perfect!

God is always right on time. How many times has God provided just what you needed, exactly when you needed it? He knows what we need at the moment we are desperate for Him to move. As we lean on His strength, God can move in ways we didn't even think of or see. You might not realize that big, whopping miracle right away, but watch out! Miracles will start happening in your life as soon as you start asking for them – from small and medium to big miracles. Each miracle is to show us that He is there and walking beside us in this journey called life.

Reflections

Is it possible for you to utter the words, "It is God's timing, not mine?"

Can you fully invest your hope and trust that God will turn your barrenness into a fertile vessel, ready for conception?

Prayer: *God, help me to trust in Your timing. Help me lay down my hopes and dreams and truly know You are doing what's best in my life. If You know my days, God, please hear my prayers. I lay my life before You now. I choose to trust in Your timing. No matter how hard it is, I will walk in faith. Amen.*

Notes:

_____

_____

_____

_____

_____

Day 15: Do You Believe?

God created man in His own image, in the image of God He created him; male and female He created them.
Genesis 1:27

*Your word is a lamp to my feet
And a light for my path.*
Psalm 119:105

The questions never seem to end, do they? In the span of a month, it's pretty clear we, as women, can think about every aspect of our lives and bodies. As we concentrate on our bodies, our fertility, and the journey, does your belief rise up in you? Do you have utter faith in God, and His plan for you, and in miracles?

Some Fertility Questions:

What does God say about you and your body?
What do you believe about yourself?
Have you thought about who you are in Christ?
Do you think this has to do with fertility?
Will pregnancy happen?
Will your family be increased?
Is ovulation happening?
Are the fallopian tubes blocked?
Is the uterus cold or hot?

Why can't I get pregnant?

Why God?

If we really believe, we declare that what the Bible says is true. We are putting our faith in the Word of God as a living truth. This truth can and should be a lamp unto our feet, guiding us through the obstacle of infertility. That's all it is, just a simple obstacle that can be overcome with prayer and faith.

God is our Shining Light

The news gets better. We are created in His image - God's perfect image. He's perfection, remember? Our bodies reflect Him. Wow, let's get excited, girls!

We can do all things through Christ who lives in us. Our thoughts can be His thoughts. Our steps are His steps. Our ways are His ways. Everything about our bodies is a mirror of God's image. The more we study the Word of God, the closer we are to becoming like Christ.

In our questions, we can turn the Word into a lamp at our feet that will light our path. He provides all the strength, solace, hope, courage, and faith we need.

Reflections

What questions do you have today for God? I choose today to believe.

I choose to know God is my shining light to conception. God is going to direct my steps perfectly.

Prayer: *I have so many questions, God, and no answers. My heart aches; my soul cries out for answers. Please, God, You are the way, the truth, and the light. I am coming to You. I need You. I need a miracle. My womb seems bare, void, and broken, kind of like my heart. But I lift my eyes up to You. Be my guiding light for this infertility journey. Show me the way. Direct me to what I need to do, if anything. I want to know I am created in Your image. So please, fix the parts that are broken, Lord. Fix me. Heal me. Amen.*

Notes:

_____

_____

_____

Day 16: True Surrender

Submit yourselves therefore to God. Resist the devil, and he will flee from you.
James 4:7

Be still, and know that I am God. I will be exalted among the nations, I will be exalted in the earth!
Psalm 56:10

I came to the end of my rope today, and my long journey to having a baby came to a screeching halt. A baby isn't, and hasn't come. It's a dark grim truth I can't ignore.

God, today I surrender the baby I can't have this month.

After seven years, I've tried it all. You would laugh if I told you all the things I've tried on this journey. Today, I realized an important truth. Nothing I've done has worked. Nothing. It's a sad reality. It's *my* reality. I've tried everything our tight budget could allow. It's funny and sad, all in the same breath. Now I can finally be honest with myself. We've come up empty.

I surrender all my failed attempts toward conception.

My hopes and dreams are never far from my thoughts and

prayers. Do you struggle with your thoughts too? It's as if your burden is never far away.

But enough is enough. For me, I have to be okay with never having a baby. I have to find peace with where I am now in my life. It is what is. I have to be able to be at peace with whatever comes my way.

I surrender my hopes and dreams.

What about you, my friend? Have you had days like mine? It's painful. It's heart-wrenching. It's abandoning our dreams and our hopes.

What you and I can cling to is supernatural faith, knowing that God is so big that He can take our broken bodies and make us healthy and fertile. That is worth a leap of faith. Faith all begins with a mustard seed. If we hold onto faith, it is critical that we surrender our entire life. When life seems at its worst, our surrender to God will give us the peace to get us through anything. The word, *surrender*, is a powerful word, which means we must yield ourselves fully to God. Wow, what a thought! Can you yield your hopes, dreams, and prayers? Can you give God your desire for a baby?

*Today, I surrender everything I am,
and everything I will be.*

I surrender all.

Our hope is that God holds us in the palms if His hands. To understand and believe this means we must trust God to know what is best for our lives. Yes, this means the how, when, and *if* we have a baby. By if, we surrender to God and trust Him, no matter what the results are. I surrender all to Jesus.

Reflections

I surrender, God. I surrender my infertility to You.

I lift my eyes to the hill where my help comes from.

Help me, God.

Prayer: *God, I choose to surrender all. I give my life to You. My life is in Your hands. Take my life, God, and do big things in me. I am desperate for a baby, but I lay my dream of a baby at Your feet. My burdens I give to You. My hopes I give to You. My sadness I give to You. I lay everything I am at the foot of the cross. God, I surrender all. Amen.*

Notes:

_____

_____

_____

_____

_____

Day 17: Fertility is my Portion

*For the LORD God is a sun and our shield.
The Lord gives grace and glory;
No good thing does He withhold from those who walk uprightly.*
Psalm 84:11

There shall be no one miscarrying or barren in your land; I will fulfill the number of your days.
Exodus 23:26

Isn't it hard to read Scriptures that say the opposite of what you feel? Maybe like me, you've had have a miscarriage, but read in Exodus where it says the opposite, "No one should have a miscarriage *or* be barren." How does this make sense? Why, God, does it say one thing, while I am living another?

The more I've thought and prayed about this, the more I've become certain of a few things:

- I am consumed with getting pregnant.
- I love caffeine more than I should.
- Exercise? Let's just say, I don't do enough.
- Ovulation is one of my top thoughts every day.
- I need lots of water I am not drinking..
- I need to pray more.
- I need to lay my burdens down.

- I stress about fertility way too much.
- I am sick of having miscarriages.

As I started thinking about me and how I cared for my body, I realized I had a greater part to play in my infertility than I ever imagined. It gave me power as I knew I could play a part in getting pregnant. What can I change about myself? How can I grow spiritually in this place? How can I line myself with God's word? God's heart doesn't want any woman to be barren. Today choose to line your hearts with God's.

Choose fertility to be your portion.

What we know for certain is God wants us to be fertile. God doesn't want us to be barren. Now, we have to get our bodies in line with the Word of God. Yes, this might mean less fast food, and zero caffeine, or lots of exercise. Maybe for you it means something different. Each of us has to look our lifestyle and see what we can change if anything.

Miscarriage doesn't have to be your portion. Choose to believe you are not barren. Accept God's blessings of fertility. Choose to believe once you have done all you can in and through your body, you must leave it in God's hands.

After eight years of trying to conceive, I have most definitely realized my steps of faith are all the things I do to make my body ready for pregnancy. After that, it's in God's hands. I must rest. I must give my infertility back to God and rest in His arms. I choose to rest.

Choose to rest in God's hands.

Today, find things you can do with your body to improve your health: exercise, vitamins, water, essential oils, etc... Once this is done, lay down your hopes and dreams. Give your fertility back to God, and let Him take charge.

I give my body to you God.

Fertility is my portion.

Infertility Tips: Whatever things you need to change, put it in prayer. Try to make decisions that both you and your spouse can do together. Take the time to talk about the changes and how they will affect you both. My goals are to drink more water; eat less fast food; and definitely do more exercise.

Reflections

What can you change to become healthier?

Can you lay your burden down and trust God to make things right?

Do you have a mustard seed of faith?

Prayer: *Let my life be a representation of You, Lord. Take my body and help me be a good steward of it. Whether it is exercise or eating healthier, help me change so that I can be fruitful and multiply. On those days when I really want my favorite soda, give me the will power to say, "No." Above anything else, please honor my heart and give us our hearts' desire.. Help us be more like You. Amen.*

Notes:

_____

_____

_____

_____

_____

Day 18: Weary and Burdened

*Come to me, all you who are weary and heavy-laden,
and I will give you rest.*
Matthew 11:28

*Cast your burden upon the Lord and He will sustain you;
He will never allow the righteous to be shaken.*
Psalm 55:22

At the end of the day, do you come home exhausted? Are you tired and weary from doing the same TTC methods month after month? If your day was like mine, I threw another negative pregnancy test away, and felt defeated. I can't seem to shake off the weariness. Yes, these are the days when the troubles of life seem to come from every direction. Can we cast those burdens to God? Now, when it's the hardest? I choose to lay down my troubles and burdens. Can you?

*God, you know what is best for me,
so I lay down my burdens in your hands.*

Ladies, when we say, "I cast my cares to You," this is the place where we find comfort. When we lay down our fears, hurts, and heartache, He will pick us back up, and give us peace. In essence, we give God the opportunity to move in our lives in ways we may not have seen or thought of. By unloading all our problems onto Him, we let Him move where He couldn't before – it's part of our letting go.

Reflections

Can you give your cares and burdens to God?

Can you trust God to help you get pregnant?

What cares do you need to put down?

Are you weary and burdened?

Never forget that God will give you rest.

He is always there, waiting to take all your burdens.

Prayer: *God I am so tired. Please help me learn to true truly surrender my worries to You. Today, I choose to lay down all my burdens: my husband, my body, our finances, our doctors, our family ...*

God, I lay every burden at Your feet. I won't pick them back up. I will wait on You and allow You to move in my life. True surrender and casting my burdens to You is my heart's desire. I long to feel the weight lifted from my shoulders. Take these burdens and move in a big way. I rest in You, God. Amen.

Notes:

Day 19: Prayer

Pray without ceasing.
1 Thessalonians 5:17

Then Hannah prayed and said,

*"My heart exults in the Lord;
My horn is exalted in the Lord,
My mouth speaks boldly against my enemies,
Because I rejoice in Your salvation.*
1 Samuel 2:1

Do you have a crazy life like mine? Finding a few moments to ourselves can be a challenge in everyday life. Whether it is work, family, or friends – finding time to focus on fertility can be its own challenge. In my house, I have essential oils, fertility teas, and often get fertility massages... Need I say more?

Anything we do in our TTC process takes time, money, and always, more patience. Finding moments for ourselves is important for us to stay grounded not only in our relationships, but every other part of our life.

Prayer brings all the parts of my life together!

Sometimes in our crazy lives, it doesn't matter what we do,

life seems to rush past us like a turbulent tornado. Before we know it, the day is over and we must look ahead to the next day.

If you can identify with me, you need a YOU moment. It could be a quick stop at a fast food joint for an icy coffee, or a massage. Find something that will work for you and your schedule. Then, take the time to make it happen.

For me, it is quiet time to pray, get acupuncture, or sip a cup of hot tea. I need thirty minutes all to myself. You better believe I utilize every second to make sure I come away feeling rejuvenated. Find that special thing you like to indulge in most. You won't regret it.

Prayer has the power to move the mountains in our lives. It may seem like we've prayed for a long time without success, but as we pray, miracles will start to happen – big and small. These miracles will give us the courage to keep going. During these times, God reminds us He is right there, walking by our side.

Reflections

Prayer can move mountains.

What prayer requests do you have? Write them down.

Prayer: *Help me pray when times are tough. Help me pray when things are good. Help me live a lifestyle of prayer so that I can really live my life walking with You. As I pray, begin doing miracles in my life. Do miracles in my husband's life. Do miracles in our bodies. Do miracles only You can do so everyone around us will see how miraculous You are. I believe. I stand strong and courageous. I walk in faith. I will pray until I see those mountains move. Then I'll start praying again. God, move our mountains. Amen.*

Notes:

_____

_____

_____

_____

_____

Day 20: Mind and Spirit Energizer

If you have been snared with the words of your mouth,
Have been caught with the words of your mouth,
Do this then, my son, and deliver yourself;
Since you have come into the hand of your neighbor,
Go, humble yourself, and importune your neighbor.
Proverbs 6:2-3

"For my thoughts are not your thoughts,
Nor are your ways My ways," declares the LORD.
Isaiah 55:8

Today, I caught myself saying I was infertile. As quickly as I said it, I stopped and said, "I am fertile. I choose fertility. I choose prosperity for my family."

Today, we will be energized by words of faith. Words of faith are the reason why I wrote this devotional. We need to speak words of life over our bodies, our marriage, and our lives.

Think about your infertility journey. Have you ever woken up in the morning and felt more tired than when you went to sleep? Exhaustion can often consume your entire being. Coffee - the decaf kind - doesn't really help. Your body seems to run on pure adrenaline. Does this sound familiar? You drag yourself through the house, ready for that Energizer moment to catapult you into a newer, and now pregnant body. Have you ever had days like that?

Words Are Powerful

Our words have the power to transform us. No matter how bad, our words set the tone for our days and our lives. We can choose to speak of life in our bodies, or stay in a cycle of complete confusion, frustration, and heartache.

You see, the Scripture is full of stories of barren women. However, God worked His miracles in each of them. I believe these stories are in the Bible for you and me to read. God knows we need to know we aren't alone. He knows how hard you and I struggle with infertility and reading about these women offers us hope and faith to believe. God is miraculous, isn't He?

Faith Walking; Faith Talking

God wants to breathe life into our bodies. We can lean on these Scriptures in the hardest days and walk in faith. We may not see it, but we can believe it - and that is faith. Find Scriptures or other "words of faith" that touch you and keep them nearby. Get yourself motivated and energized; our days can be strengthened by taking steps of faith.

Reflections

Did you know that God's Word is our daily energizer?

Find a Scripture or word of faith to memorize today.

Prayer: *God, make me into Your image. I need my body to work properly. I speak in faith believing that You will make my ovaries, my fallopian tubes, and every other part of my body work correctly. I am fertile. Thank You for making me fertile. Change my thoughts and prayers. Breathe life into my body. As I struggle with getting pregnant, move big in my life. I need to start each day energized. I need to have hope, God. Give me the words to say. Give me the prayers to pray at the exact moment I need them. Help me walk by faith. Move big in my life, God. Amen.*

Notes:

_____

_____

_____

_____

_____

Day 21: True Love

*"How beautiful you are, my darling,
How beautiful you are!
Your eyes are like doves."
"How handsome you are, my beloved,
And so pleasant!
Indeed, our couch is luxuriant!"*
Song of Solomon 1:15-16

Have you read the Song of Solomon lately? Shut the front door! You have got to close out the world and get ready for romance galore! This book is all about true love. No matter what day you ovulate, pull this one out as you approach your fertile days. Get yourself pumped up and ready, because you are going to love this!

True Love: Love is in the air today. What more can I say? It is all about love, romance, and "the kisses of his mouth." Today it is all about kisses, love, and sweet nothings. If you aren't sure what sweet nothings are, just remember that time your spouse whispered into your ear, and you immediately started giggling – that, my friends, was a sweet nothing.

Sweet Nothings = Romance

Although we don't always think of the Bible as being a how-to for romance, it is certainly that. The Scriptures can really help us with every problem we have, including desire! I challenge you to read up on marriage and romance straight from the Bible. Not only do we get a passionately clear idea of the true meaning of what our relationship should be, but we also see romantic stories that could be the basis for the best chick flick, I guess, but let me backtrack.

How often do you go on dates?

Marriage and romance should go hand in hand, but sometimes we get so caught up in life, with work, family, and the biggest one of all… drum roll, please… Trying to Get Pregnant! Some might think that trying to get pregnant should be simultaneous with passion, but after so long, well, ladies, give me an Amen if you get my meaning…

Take a Moment to Reflect on Your Journey.

Remember way, way back when? You know what I'm talking about. That day your heart did a somersault every time your true love walked into the room when you were first dating?

I remember that day like it was yesterday. I can't help but remember how I felt as it's forever engraved in my memory. Oh my, I was head over heels in love. I think I hear a song in my head… and it's like true love all over again.

Do you remember that first kiss? It seemed to be in slow motion. It was THE kiss. I remember the day, the hour, the feeling… Oops! Getting carried away in my own memories… Let me get back to the subject, ladies. I tend to get lost in my own thoughts when I speak about my husband.

The point is: we all know how hectic life can be. I mean,

trying to get pregnant can become a tedious, OCD-like cycle that doesn't seem to ever end. It's like a revolving door and we can't seem to find our way out. It's that scary roller coaster that goes on forever. The truth is that infertility is like an evil word when we are trying to keep the romance alive. If life weren't easy before, it becomes a hundred percent harder.

Who has time to remember how if felt to be like giddy teenagers? Our lives change over time. Our marriages change. Bills happen. Work stinks. And problems arise.

No matter how long you've been married, there is always time for a whisper, kiss, a hug, a touch, or a promise of what will come later. We have to make romance a priority. We must make time for romance!

We can and should stay in the honeymoon phase forever. No matter how much life changes, our connection with our spouses will carry us through the hardest of times. I'm not joking. Hearing the promise of later years can turn the darkest day into a time of hope.

Now, you don't have to be like me and scream from the church softball game bleachers, "I love my hottie husband!" What a shock that was for the other church-going baseball enthusiasts! What was once shock, however, has since turned into playful teasing and expectation from the players. They expect it from me now because I am all about my husband and have been since the day we married.

I am a wife who LOVES her husband.

That feeling keeps me sane during the difficult moments.

Romance is like a chick flick that should never end. Basically, we need these romantic moments to keep our love fresh and new. Infertility and trying to conceive with infertility issues can be excruciatingly difficult on you, your spouse, and your marriage. In these times, each of us needs extra romance.

Romance is VITAL for a successful marriage.

We need those secluded moments that break down the burdens we all feel. Romance could be holding hands, sitting on the couch, or having a date. Sometimes, it is just as simple as it is complex. Do whatever works for you.

Romance helps us de-stress from the chaotic flow of our lives. It doesn't always happen naturally, ladies. We have to make time. Yep, each of us has to put in the hard work if we want to see the fantastic results.

Infertility Tips: Find what works for you. Perhaps your husband brings you home a surprise just because he loves you. Surprise him with a toe-clenching, mouthwatering kiss that will knock his socks off. That's the way we smolder the fire. Don't just use a tiny match; let's douse it with lighter fluid! Whoosh! Keep your husband surprised!

Reflections

Take your love on the most passionate ride of your life.

Try new things.

Pray together.

Kiss a lot.

Encourage each other.

Love each other.

    Prayer: *Give my marriage a splash of romance. Let all our worries and stress fall away until all we have left is each other. I want romance, God. I need romance. I want my husband to see me, hold me, and love me. I want to feel his love. I want to be there for him. Help us turn to each other in the moment's stress. Help us see each other instead of the problems. Help us rely on each other on the good and bad days. Help us keep the romance alive and strong. Help me become selfless. Help me be bold. I will be bold. I will do the unexpected. Help me, Father God. Amen.*

Notes:

_____

_____

Day 22: Jealousy

You lust and do not have; so you commit murder. You are envious and cannot obtain; so you fight and quarrel. You do not have because you do not ask. You ask and do not receive, because you ask with wrong motives, so that you may spend it on your pleasures.
James 4:2-3

Jealousy, my friends, is brutal to each of us. It can eat away at your beautiful heart and demeanor. Instead of peace, we feel jealousy. The jealousy then turns to anger, and the anger to bitterness. If we are truthful, we experience many emotions, each more difficult than the one before.

To overcome this vicious cycle, let's go back to the beginning. Think about the moment you see a lady with the very thing you want: a baby. What do you feel in that moment?

Pain, Jealousy, and Grief

Are these the emotions you felt? If so, you are not alone. The one feeling that can drop us to our knees in pain is jealousy. In order to overcome this strong emotion, sometimes you and I have to do the impossible. Bless those mothers. Pray for them. Serve them. Do for them as you would want for yourself.

A heart at peace gives life to the body,

but envy rots the bones.

A heart at peace is what every woman struggling with infertility needs and deserves. When we apply this Scripture, we will see and experience blessings. Yes, you may still hurt. Yes, the grief might still be there. The more we can bless, the more blessings will come back to us. Yes, we might still struggle with infertility. The journey may not be over.

But you will feel the blessing!

The truth is: it might be painful to serve the people who have what you crave: a baby. Yes, you might have crying moments. Yes, you might ache. If you can be courageous and bless them still, you will reap the blessings. As you bless those mothers, there isn't room for other emotions. Little by little, the jealousy will begin to diminish and no longer vex you. It is worth trying to see the results in your life.

Jacqueline's Journal:
One year, I went through five pregnancies, five baby showers, and five hospital visits. I was at my wit's end. To add insult to injury, I was also the birthing coach to a young lady. Talk about sacrifice! In my sorrow, I served others. In my service, the blessings came. In the blessings, I found peace. In the peace, I found hope.

My time will come, and your time will come.

When you are faced with pregnant women, another baby shower, or another birth, and you feel lost in the depths of despair, pray for the people who have what you want. Bless them. Serve them. Encourage them.

It feels good to bless others.

Reflections

Today is a great day to focus on others, bless others, and encourage others.

Prayer: *Oh Lord, I can't stop the jealousy as I watch the same cycle over and over. My heart is overwhelmed with grief. Why, God? Why does everyone else get pregnant but me? Please God, help me to lay aside jealousy and bless those around me. Help me serve in my greatest sorrow. Help me overcome my jealousy. Teach me to be selfless. God, I need Your help. I can't walk this journey alone. Amen.*

Notes:

_____

_____

_____

_____

_____

Day 23: Selfishness -- Not Me?

*He who separates himself seeks his own desires,
He quarrels against all sound wisdom.*
Proverbs 18:1

Infertility can strike the heart of a woman. Whether it's the inability to conceive or the disappointment of our bodies not working properly, it's normal to feel very strong emotions. Maybe, that's even putting it mildly for how we really feel.

What about our spouses? Do you think they go through the same emotions as you? Well, the answer is: most have mixed emotions:

   1. No, they can't feel what women go through.
   2. Yes, they go through the same emotions as us.
   3. Heck, no! They can't understand what women go through.

Sadly, this is a tough devotional for me as it hits me right down to my very quick. For way too long, I've treated my husband as if he didn't understand. How could he? Cramps, periods, blood clots, miscarriages, more pain.... The list could go on and on. He doesn't understand how my body works. He doesn't feel the pain I have to endure.

Maybe they doesn't understand those exact things, but your spouse and mine have been walking right by our sides through it all. Although they can't understand our true emotions, we can't understand theirs either.

All too often, it's easy for life to be all about us. We are the ones going through the conception attempts, after all. And we are the ones enduring the miscarriages. For me, it was after many heated conversations with my husband that I saw the light.

I, Jacqueline Winslow (put in your own name), was selfish. I had become an all-about-me-kind-of-person. Instead of pregnancy being about us, it had become all about me.

The truth was: my handsome husband hurt as badly as I did. He ached for a baby just like me. He grieved for the baby we lost just like me. And he cried just like me.

Reflections

My husband often deserves more credit than I give him. Can you relate?

He understands the pain because he is walking by my side throughout this journey.

I choose to stop being selfish.

I choose to think about my husband's feelings instead of my own through this infertility journey.

Prayer: *God, help me look past myself. Help me to be selfless. In my pain, God help me turn my eyes to You. I choose to put my husband first and be attentive to his needs. God help me. Help me look past my own pain to see my spouse's pain as well. I need You, God. I can't do this alone. Change me. Amen.*

Notes:

_____

_____

_____

Day 24: Hannah's Prayer

"I am Hannah"

Then Hannah rose after eating and drinking in Shiloh. Now Eli the priest was sitting on the seat by the doorpost of the temple of the L<small>ORD</small>.
She, greatly distressed, prayed to the L<small>ORD</small> and wept bitterly.
She made a vow and said, "O L<small>ORD</small> of hosts, if You will indeed look on the affliction of Your maidservant and remember me, and not forget Your maidservant, but will give Your maidservant a son, then I will give him to the L<small>ORD</small> all the days of his life, and a razor shall never come on his head."
Now it came about, as she continued praying before the L<small>ORD</small>, that Eli was watching her mouth.
As for Hannah, she was speaking in her heart, only her lips were moving, but her voice was not heard. So Eli thought she was drunk. Then Eli said to her, "How long will you make yourself drunk? Put away your wine from you."
But Hannah replied, "No, my lord, I am a woman oppressed in spirit; I have drunk neither wine nor strong drink, but I have poured out my soul before the L<small>ORD</small>.
Do not [e]consider your maidservant as a worthless woman, for I have spoken until now out of my great concern and provocation."
Then Eli answered and said, "Go in peace; and may the God of Israel grant your petition that you have asked of Him." She said, "Let your maidservant find favor in your sight." So the woman went her way and ate, and her face was no longer sad.

Samuel 1:9-20

Is your journey anything like Hannah's? It is if you are like me, and I've reread this Scripture more times than I can count. Although my husband doesn't have more than one wife, (thank goodness!) I can attest to being barren.

The truth is: I just haven't been able to stay pregnant. No matter how hard I try. I've done everything, yes, ladies, and that includes every old wives' tale you've ever heard. Boy, do I have home remedy stories I could tell…

Do you have a Hannah story?

Hannah was a woman just like you and me. She saw women around her having babies that even included another wife! – talk about us having problems, she had MAJOR problems! When I think about how much I've cried in my private sanctuary (ahem, the bathroom), I can't imagine the rivers of tears she wept. She also lived through our pain.

This woman is a hero to every woman struggling to get pregnant. In her worst hour, she cried out to the Lord. She turned her desperate tears into a prayer that still resonates for you and me.

"And she made a vow, saying, *'LORD Almighty, if you will only look on your servant's misery and remember me, and not forget your servant but give her a son, then I will give him to the LORD for all the days of his life, and no razor will ever be used on his head."*

This is a prayer like no other.

Prayer: *Remember me, Lord. Don't forget your servant. Give me a son. This son you give me, I'll give him back to you so he can serve you all the days of your life. Oh, God, Remember me.*

Jacqueline's Journal

As I write this, I can't stop the tears. Ladies, this plea hits home for me. This is my prayer. This is your prayer. This is my journey. You and I are living Hannah's infertility journey. We understand her pain. We can embrace her jealousy and envy. We have empathy for her. We feel her heartbreak as she cried out to God, yet again. Because we all know this wasn't the first time she prayed.

Prayer, for a barren or infertile woman, just comes with the territory. We know prayer. We live prayer.

Desperation Often Brings Us to Our Knees in Prayer

In our desperation, we go to our Heavenly Father, feeling so desperate for a miracle, we would do anything. Anything! For Hannah, she promised to give her son back to God, if He would just give her a son!

If I were there, I would have said, "Enough already, God. I need a baby. I need a son. I'll do anything to have one!" And she did. She was desperate for a baby just like you and I are.

Guess what? God answered her prayer! Not only granting her a pregnancy, but also allowing her to give birth to a baby boy, Samuel. God answered every last detail. And she followed through with her promise too. Oh, this woman was a true hero.

Hannah's legacy gives us hope. She reminds us that God loves the little children. He loves us and cares about the details. He loves you! He doesn't speak about barrenness, but about life. He speaks of life over you this very second. Let the following prayer soak into you as you kneel in desperation. I love this prayer.

Reflections

It's nearly impossible to read this story without being moved, shaken, and faith-driven.

If God did it for Hannah, he can do it for you! Hold onto this Bible story; and read it often.

Prayer: *Remember me, Lord. Don't forget your servant. Give me a son. This son You give me, I'll give him back to You so he can serve You all the days of his life. Give me a daughter. This daughter You give me, I'll give her back to You so she can serve You all the days of her life. I will train him or her in the Christ-like ways that they should live. I will be a good steward of these gifts. Oh, God, remember me. Amen.*

Notes:

_____

_____

_____

_____

_____

Day 25: An "I Can" Attitude

I can do all things through Him who strengthens me.
Philippians 4:13

On emotional days, it is hard to believe we can do all things like ovulation, pregnancy, communication, romance, marriage, work, and every other situation you may be dealing with in your life.

When life gets hard, do you find yourself on an emotional roller coaster? If so, you have two choices: either walk in the discouragement of the circumstance, or walk in faith.

Admittedly, each of us has tried NOT to walk in the traumatic circumstance we may find ourselves in. As Christians, we are commanded to walk in faith and not by sight. Ever feel like you don't have enough faith for whatever situation you are going through? If so, you aren't alone. God knows we have moments like those, so he gave us the Scriptures, just for such moments.

I can do all things through Christ who strengthens me.

We can do all things, *all things!* I'll confess, ladies. Thinking I will never get pregnant has slipped in my thoughts more times than I can count. Then I look at this Scripture and I have to smack my own hand. Shame on me! I can do it. I know I can do it because I can; and you can too. We can do all things through Christ who strengthens us. Pregnancy is our portion!

No matter what situation you and I must face, having an "I

can" attitude often changes our entire demeanor. Isn't it amazing that we can actually alter our circumstances just by what we say and do? Try to say "I can" rather than "I can't."

We CAN do ALL things through Christ who gives us the strength each time we struggle! He is right in the middle of the toughest situations! He won't let you down.

Reflections

You can make it through anything with God beside you.

You CAN and WILL make it.

What situations in your life do you need to remind yourself you can and will make it?

Prayer: *God, today I lift up my eyes to the hill where my help comes from. You are my help. Help me to believe, in the moment, that I can do all things through You who strengthens us. When I'm down, I choose to believe. I choose to lift up my eyes. I choose to believe that I can do anything, with You walking beside me. I need to feel Your presence around me as I go about my day. Today, I choose to trust in You and know that I can do anything with You by my side. Thank you, for the Scriptures which sustain me on days when I feel hopeless. I love You, God. Amen.*

Notes:

_____

_____

_____

Day 26: Cramping Prayer

Pray without ceasing.
1 Thessalonians 5:17

And the Lord will take away from you all sickness, and will affect you with none of the terrible diseases of Egypt which you have known, but will lay them on all those who hate you.
Deuteronomy 7:15

I hate cramping. Don't you? Do you consider it the harbinger of what is about to come? I know instantly, after that very first cramp, once again, I'm not pregnant.

Cramping can suck the life right out of you. It hurts physically and mentally. This is when we must turn to prayer. Prayer is the act of talking to God. Talk to Him like you would another person. Know this: when you start praying, especially in the throes of desperation, it can and will change your life.

Miracles happen when we pray. Mountains are moved.

When we encounter the obstacles in our life, sometimes, prayer is the only thing we have left. We feel hopeless, powerless, and spent emotionally. Prayer can alert the angels on our behalf. We need prayer, and we need to pray. Prayers can change everything. This, I know, and I live it out in my own life. Your prayers are real. God hears every one of them.

Every person struggling with infertility faces many of the same hurdles. Our hearts get wrenched in the same ways. I quote here a page from my own infertility journal.

Jacqueline's Journal
I feel it coming: cramping, headaches, leg aches, stomach pain, and the all-out emotional roller coaster. I know the signs and symptoms that usually mean I'm once again NOT pregnant. My heart, yet again, aches for the one thing that seems to always elude me: pregnancy. Why me? Why not me?

Today, I feel depleted. All I have, and all I know to do, is pray. Let this prayer be what God wanted for today. Today, He is working in me, changing me, molding me. God will surely create a benefit for having to endure another month of not getting pregnant. He makes all things possible.

God, heal me. Touch my body. Heal these cramps. Help me choose to focus on the positive today. Amen.

Yes, our pain is real, but it doesn't matter how bad it gets, we can still fall on our knees and begin praying. We may not understand, and we may not agree with God's ways. We can talk to Him. We can lift up our eyes to the source of all help. When we have nothing left inside us, we can pray. We can always pray.

Reflections

Write down a prayer to keep handy for those days when you just feel terrible. On the days when I have nothing left, I refer to the infertility prayers I've already written. I manage to find the words to say even when I have no words left.

Prayer: *God, help me to have hope and faith. Help me to stay strong on days like today. Give me the courage to begin each day new and fresh. I choose to praise You, God, no matter what I feel. I choose to lift my eyes up to You and I will praise You whether I get pregnant this month or not. I praise Your holy name, especially when my spirit is downcast. You are faithful.*

I pour out my heart to You, Father God, because You are faithful. Oh God, I know I can conceive because my body is working well enough to have a period. Touch me. Heal whatever isn't working properly. With each tear that falls down my face, I choose to trust that You know what is best for me. Please give me a miracle. Thank You for always being by my side. I love You, God. I revere Your holy name. Amen

Notes:

_____

_____

Day 27: Spread the Love

The things which you have heard from me in the presence of many witnesses, entrust these to faithful men who will be able to teach others also.
2 Timothy 2:2

> *Follow Jesus.*
>
> *Be Christ-like.*
>
> *Tell your story to others.*
>
> *How simple is that?*

Let's break it down, ladies. It is vital to share what we've learned with others. There are ladies struggling with infertility, limited finances, marriages, children, and every other subject under the sun. We live complex lives and face diverse problems every day. There are women right now who need to hear about your experiences. Remember that Scripture that always lifts you up? Share it. You have undergone hardships and uncomfortable situations AND you've learned to deal in ways that could help others.

Think about this: when someone tells you a story, does it often remind you of one of your own? This could apply to fertility, infertility, miscarriages, conception, and even pregnancy. All women have stories to tell. We love to tell our journeys and stories, don't we? I do. What about you?

Use your knowledge to empower others.

If you observe a young woman crying, after trying to get pregnant for three months without success, you just might have the key to her successful pregnancy. Use your struggles and achievements to help others. Sadly, the pain you and I have endured is just another opportunity to bless someone.

Our Life Messes are Huge Opportunities

If there is one thing I've discovered through my own infertility, it's that many women are impeded in their attempts to get pregnant. I know; isn't that a *duh* statement? It doesn't matter if they've failed for three months and are still not sure what they're doing wrong, or tried to conceive for years.

Women need hope!

You and I can give others hope when we channel our pain and disappointment into blessing others. You might have an ovulation tip that could be a life-changer. Or, maybe you found a prayer that helps you every time a particularly sad situation happens. Your voice could even change someone's life.

Reflections

Find someone to share your journey with. Share the miracles God has performed in your life.

Share all your infertility remedies that work!

You have special knowledge that others need to hear!

Prayer: *Help me be aware of the women around me. Help me be sensitive to their needs. No matter what is going on with my day, help me be selfless. Help me share my story, even when it's hard. Especially when it's painful, give me opportunities to share. Help me encourage others by using my life as a testimony. Give me miracles so I can share with others what You have done in my life. Amen.*

Notes:

_____

_____

_____

_____

_____

Day 28: "Life Messes"

Now on the last day, the great day of the feast, Jesus stood and cried out, saying, "If anyone is thirsty, let him come to Me and drink.
John 7:37

Draw near to God and He will draw near to you. Cleanse your hands, you sinners; and purify your hearts, you double-minded.
James 4:8

    Isn't it amazing to know there is a river of life that God wants to have flowing through us? He is always there for us. His river of life provides hope, strength, encouragement, perseverance, patience, and kindness. Okay, you get the drift. Whatever you need, He will become that.

River of life, come flow through us!

If we believe in Him, the stream of living water will flow effortlessly through you and me. It doesn't matter what you need, He will be there; and the more you believe, the more miracles will happen for you. Now that is good news! As we go through life, we will eventually encounter what I fondly like to call "life messes." Things happen. Life happens. It can stink sometimes. In my life, when one bad thing happens, it just seems to spiral downward from there. I've seen it over and over again. You'd think I would have learned the lesson! I'm what I like to call a slow learner. How about you?

What do you do when things begin to spiral out of control? What is your first go-to emotion? Are you distraught? Out of control? Frustrated? Irritated? All of those emotions are understandable. Let's face it; we all have that one emotion at the hint of a "life mess." Maybe, there is something better.

These "life messes" are actually opportunities. Yes, opportunities. Each time something goes wrong, we have a choice to walk in faith or throw a pity party. I've done both, so there are no accusations here, just an undeniable truth.

God never leaves us or forsakes us, no matter what the "life mess" is. However, knowing and living in Him are quite another matter. I know, it sounds all good until we
apply it. If we choose to dwell in His river of life, well, guess what? We reap the rewards.

But if we choose to wallow in self-pity (Yep, I've done that), well, then, we miss out. We miss out greatly. The hardest part is that God gives us the choice. We can choose to rely on Him, or ourselves. We must choose.

Tips to overcoming life messes:

- Control your thoughts
- Read the Scriptures
- Choose to NOT think about your life mess
- Listen to Christian music
- Quote Scriptures
- Memorize Scriptures
- Remember God's promise.

- Pray with your spouse
- Have quiet time

If you are a prayer warrior (like me), you know that praying is one way of attracting that river of life and making it flow through you. We crave it. We want to be ever closer to God. Yet, when those "life messes" happen, it's all too easy to revert back to our old ways of life – Letting Our Emotions Rule Our Situations.

The more we depend on God, the less we depend on ourselves. In our infertility struggles, we need God's hand on our lives. If we turn to Him as the infertility situations arise, He will be there. Now, *that* is growth, my friends.

God is always there, waiting for us. His peace is right there and ours for the taking. This means, there's no room for doubt or frustration. In God, we can do anything.

Reflections

When you feel yourself spiraling out of control, choose to depend on God.

Ask God what you should do in your "life messes."

Prayer: *Oh God, this is so fresh on my heart. So many life messes" surround me. Each time, tears of frustration are my first response. God, I choose You. I choose to focus on You. You are my rock, my shield, and my strength. You can do anything. So I wait on You. I will choose not to focus on my situation. I will choose to walk in faith and not by sight. You can use these uncomfortable situations for good. I choose to believe that You are going to use them for good. Use me. Help me control my thoughts, my emotions, and my words. My life messes will not control me. Through You, anything is possible. Amen.*

Notes:

_____

_____

_____

_____

_____

Day 29: Dark Tunnel of Heartbreak

He heals the brokenhearted and binds up their wounds.
Psalms 147:3

*The righteous cry, and the L*ORD *hears*
And delivers them out of all their troubles.
*The L*ORD *is near to the brokenhearted*
And saves those who are crushed in spirit.
Many are the afflictions of the righteous,
*But the L*ORD *delivers him out of them all.*
He keeps all his bones,
Not one of them is broken.
Psalms 34:17-20

Jacqueline's Journal

I'm right in the midst of the dark tunnel today. Have you had a day like this? It's a feeling of total heartbreak at your doorstep? The rain falls and doesn't seem to let up? The pain is real. It seems so dark and empty all around me. This tunnel is a roller coaster of sadness. My tunnel is my journey, and it is so vivid and real before me. A cruel heartache rips through me.

God is great.

Does today's journal entry resonate with you? This entry is a vivid picture of any day in the life of a woman dealing with infertility. They come often.

He is a great God.

My heart is aching. The internal turmoil hasn't gone away. For once, I just don't know what to do. I look over at my husband; he's in the same place. We just feel lost. We stare at each other with looks of complete confusion. Why, God? Why?

Praise The Lord, Oh, My Soul.

I can't seem to find the strength to pray. I can't even think straight. My head hurts from crying. It feels like we're the only ones. Are we the only ones struggling to have a child, God? Are we the only ones who can't seem to get our prayers answered? Are we? I'm tired, God. I'm tired of crying out. My strength is gone. I feel completely depleted.

God, I need You now.

It's dark outside, and I don't know why, but it always seems worse when it's dark. Maybe it's times like this when we only have ourselves, our thoughts, and of course, our unanswered prayers.

As I sit here listening to my favorite Christian music, I can't help but wonder, *why me?* Does God have some special plan I don't know about? What is it, God? What do You want from me? I didn't choose this path. In fact, I never dreamed we'd be here.

Why should we? We're a young, fit, happily married couple. We were excited to start planning a family - seven years later, and we're still trying. Oh God! My heart cries out for something, *anything* good to happen!

God, take our pain away.

Questions can haunt us, and we all have them. God never said he would answer all our endless questions, but I wish He would. However, He promised He would walk through our trials with us. We are never alone.

If you've also asked questions of God, without receiving answers, the truth is, we may never know the reason why. But know this: when we are in the worst of the worse, it's vital that we lift up our eyes, dry our tears, and raise our voices up to heaven. The answers and our ultimate freedom lie in our praise and faith. We may not know why life presents such trials, but in our heartache, our praise can and will lift us out of any turbulent situation.

Our trials allow us the privilege to love God despite whatever comes our way. Sometimes, ladies, it's a downright difficult journey. When we are heartbroken, afraid, and feeling hopeless, this is when we need to put our trust in Him. He will give us strength! This is honest-to-goodness real! Only He can bring us out of the tunnel. Why and how?

He's a great God.

No matter what we must endure, we have the assurance, if we look beyond our predicaments, and focus on Him, that freedom will come. Peace will again reign in our hearts. Our

Savior died so we could have life. He will always work on our behalf.

We aren't alone. Sure, we may be experiencing trials, but it's just a great opportunity for God to move in a big way. Who needs miracles? I do. I can and will praise Him.

Reflections

No matter what comes your way, choose Him.

Choose Him and you will reap the rewards.

Some days are just plain difficult, yet we can choose to praise Him despite it all.

Prayer: *Move in a big way, God. We need You to come. I need You, in a big way, God. My trials aren't getting smaller. My heart is aching for something, anything to happen. I need You to move in my life. I need You to move in a powerful way. Amen.*

Notes:

_____

_____

_____

_____

_____

Day 30: Overcoming Miscarriage

*Come to Me, all who are weary and heavy-laden,
and I will give you rest. Take My yoke upon you and learn
from Me, for I am gentle and humble in heart,
and you will find rest for your souls.*
Matthew 11:28-29

*For Your righteousness, O God, reaches to the heavens,
You who have done great things;
O God, who is like You?
You who have shown me many troubles and distresses
Will revive me again,
And will bring me up again from the depths of the earth.
May You increase my greatness
And turn to comfort me.*
Psalm 71:19-21

Miscarriage…

*How can we prepare for a miracle and then
endure such heartbreak?*

When miscarriage happens, what next?

My heart is broken – what now, God?

How's that for an intro? I must be honest. I cry every time I read this chapter. Before I begin, I have to warn you. Be prepared to cry. Be prepared to enter a place that is very scary.

Be prepared to be honest. Be prepared to think about the little baby that is now in heaven.

Jacqueline's First Miscarriage

The day was dark, cloudy even. Yet inside, I was leaping for joy. I was pregnant. God answered our prayers! For days and weeks my heart was in a whirlwind of anticipation. Our prayers were answered. Everything we prayed for was now a reality.

Three months later, I felt what can only be described as my heart crumbling. I knew the very second it happened. I lost the baby. Tears poured down my cheeks as I made my way to the bathroom. *No! Oh God, not now! Just when we had our miracle!* My tears were real. My heart was in agonizing devastation as we drove to the doctor's office only to hear what I already knew. Our baby was gone.

After losing our baby through miscarriage, I had no idea how many emotions I would go through. I was up, I was down, and in a matter of seconds. The sadness didn't seem to go away. I couldn't staunch the heartache, or lessen the sheer pain inside my soul.

I learned in those moments that walking in faith and not by sight was NOT easy. Especially after we just received our big miracle - then our eagerly anticipated baby was gone.

In our darkest place, we clung together. We allowed each other the right to have emotions, and we gave each other space. Crazy how you can cling to one another and give space, but that is exactly what we did. In those first hours, we didn't understand. There was no way to understand, nor did we try to hide the grief we felt.

As I stood in the hospital, crying uncontrollably, I chose to believe in God and His ultimate plan for us. I just had a miscarriage. "God I trust in you." I just lost my baby. "God I trust you will work all things for good." This is where it gets real. If I am going to live my life as a Christian, I have to believe He works all things for good, and I have to walk it out. And I did, in the hardest day of my life.

We can't always understand His ways. We don't have to. We just have to trust in Him. You see, God didn't promise we wouldn't have more obstacles to overcome. Simply put, life isn't always peaches and cream. This, you and I know already too well.

What we can count on is that as each day passes, every time we lifted our eyes to Him, the pain subsided just a little more. Sure, we went through the grieving process. It may take a long time. It may take a long time, but we will get through it. We will make it. We will try again.

As my husband and I lifted our eyes on god, we found we had the strength to get through that difficult season. Whatever storm you face, You will make it through any storm too. Find a Christian song that touches you and listen to it as often as you need. I've had one special song on repeat more times than I can count. Do whatever you can to find peace.

Lift up your hands to heaven and release your little one to God. He's a great God. He will look over your little baby because He's our Father. We can trust in Him.

Reflections

God will be there on the darkest of days. Sometimes all we can say is, "It *will* be well with my soul."

Prayer: *Father God, I choose to release my baby (the baby's name) to You. I choose to believe that You know best. You created the heavens and the stars. You knew the daylight needed the sun and the evening needed the moon. God, You planned every hair on our heads. You are our Creator. You are our Father. Take our baby and thank You for giving us the gift we had for the brief time we had him (or her). Now it's time for us to release our pain, and our heartache, into Your hands. Let us find healing. Amen.*

Notes:

_____

_____

_____

_____

_____

Continuing Story:
The second miscarriage just happened. I didn't have enough time to publish this devotional before I was back to where we started. The grief was overwhelming. The heartache – well, there aren't words.

This miscarriage, losing a second baby, was harder than the first miscarriage. Our faith, hope and trust seemed shattered as soon as we found out we miscarried again. I held our little baby in my hands, and we stared in disbelief and agony. Somehow, God lifted us up, and held us tight. I knew it. I felt His arms around me.

YOU ARE NOT ALONE!

God was with us every second, every minute, and every hour in that hospital room. The darkest day, and yet, God was there. I felt Him all around me.

Through it all, the little nugget of hope that carried us beyond our grief was the realization we could get pregnant. It finally happened again. After several years of nothing, it actually, finally happened. Yes, we lost our little angel, but hope prevailed and somehow, we were able to hang onto God's promise. It happened for us. Yes, our story will continue…

The third miscarriage was far worse than the first or the second. The pain, the emotions, the hospital visit, the heartbreak; it created a horror movie that I can replay over and over in my mind.
I choose to lay down that night in the hands of God.

I choose to let God's comfort surround me, cover me.
I choose to release my little one back to heaven.

Have you ever cried out to the God of Heavens and wondered if he had forgotten you? That was what our third miscarriage was like. The tears, the cry out for help, yet the baby did pass. We did have a miscarriage at the hospital.

As I look back at that night, even as we drove to the hospital, the very truth is that God *was* with us. The pain was so deep, so crushing, at the time I know I questioned, "God are you here?"

But God was there.

He did not leave of forsake us.

Even now, I don't understand the how's or why's. The crushing moment the baby falls into your hands. The sheer panic when I look up at my husband then back down at the little mass that was our baby. There are no answers to that kind of moment. As I held the little baby in my hands, time stood still for a second. There are no words for that kind of moment. Only sheer grief can describe those moments. The grief that only His grace can cover us through ... His Grace can and did help us make it through those dark moments.

God's Grace is Sufficient

Reflections

Our little ones are in heaven. The angels are rejoicing. Their time in the heavens is just the beginning for them.

We will focus on the good, and try again. We will definitely try again.

It WILL be well with my soul. It will, as long as I have faith. I choose faith, now in this moment.

Can you say this during the crisis? Can you believe in faith that it will be well with your soul?

Prayer: *God, meet us at this place. Be near. Hold us close. Lift us up out of this place. Restore our faith. Give us renewed hope. Help me believe it will be well with my soul. Amen.*

Notes:

_____

_____

_____

_____

_____

Day 31: Infertility Prayer

Pray, then, in this way:

'Our Father who is in heaven,
Hallowed be Your name.
'Your kingdom come.
Your will be done,
On earth as it is in heaven.
'Give us this day our daily bread.
'And forgive us our debts, as we also have forgiven our debtors.
'And do not lead us into temptation, but deliver us from evil. For Yours is the kingdom and the power and the glory forever. Amen.
Matthew 6:9-13

Jacqueline's Infertility Prayer

Dear Lord, I come to You as Your humble servant. I live my life as a testimony of Your goodness. You have been faithful in my life, and I thank You. In the morning I praise You. In the evening I praise You. I will continue to praise for You are faithful.

Today, my Father God, I come to You with a special request. I need You to move mightily in my body. Your Word says you speak life over me. You speak life over my womb. Your Word says that You love the little children. God, I need to feel that love. I need to see Your supernatural miracles in my life and body. I've prayed for big and small miracles throughout my infertility journey, and I've seen countless miracles. God, I need big miracles. I need Hannah-sized miracles. Send the rain into my life, my body, and my finances. My husband and I need to see You move so we can share with others how miraculous You are. Oh, God, this is my prayer. I love You with all my heart. I want to seek Your ways. I want my life to reflect You. But my heart is crying out because my soul grieves for what I can't have. In my sorrow, I lift my eyes up to the hill where my help comes from. As I lift my eyes up to You, I lay these burdens at Your feet. Amen.

What is your prayer?

_____

_____

_____

_____

_____

_____

_____

Dear Friend,

Although we've concluded a full month of devotions, sadly, for many of us, it starts over again in the next month. We start each month new and fresh, somehow reminding ourselves that God is still on the throne. He IS working on our behalf. Somehow. Someway. He will finish what he started in us. Our wombs will be healthy, whole, and full of life. Let's have faith together!

God *will* work all the highs and lows of our infertility journey for good.

With love and prayers,
Jacqueline Winslow
www.infertilitystinks.com

May God bless each of us with the cries of our hearts.
May we find faith to walk through each of our situations.
May God give us mercies to deal with every "life mess" that comes our way! Most of all, please God, perform miracles for every person who reads this book. Let my life, my screw-ups, and my infertility be an example and a guide to comfort and encourage others.
Amen.

Just for laughs...

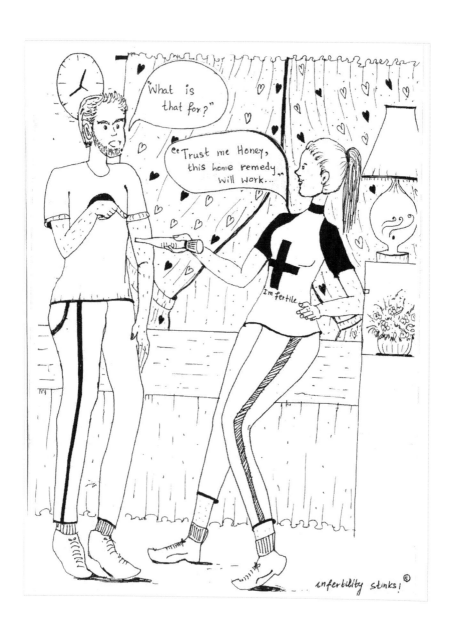

Books by Jacqueline Winslow

Infertility Stinks! A 31 Day Devotional

If you love Christian romance, be sure to check out:

***No Time for Love* Short Story #1 of Roanoke True Love**
(Kindle Only)

More Than We Bargained For (Kindle Only)

Made in the USA
Las Vegas, NV
09 June 2022